Yoga Teacher Planner

   Name : ______________________

   Address: ______________________

   Phone: ______________________

   Email: ______________________

Yoga Teacher Planner

Date

Time

Venue

Theme/Focus:

Props

Oils

Music

No. Of Attendees:

Private class: y / n

Note

Feedback

☆ ☆ ☆ ☆ ☆

Mantra / Positive Quote:

Yoga Teacher Planner

Date

Time

Venue

Theme/Focus:

Props

Oils

Music

No. Of
Attendees:

Private class: y / n

Note

○
○
○
○
○
○
○
○

Feedback

☆ ☆ ☆ ☆ ☆

Mantra / Positive Quote:

Yoga Teacher Planner

Date

Time

Venue

Theme/Focus:

Props

Oils

Music

No. Of Attendees:

Private class: y / n

Note

Feedback

☆ ☆ ☆ ☆ ☆

Mantra / Positive Quote:

Yoga Teacher Planner

Date

Time

Venue

Theme/Focus:

Props

Oils

Music

No. Of
Attendees:

Private class: y / n

Note

○

○

○

○

○

○

○

○

Feedback

☆ ☆ ☆ ☆ ☆

Mantra / Positive Quote:

Yoga Teacher Planner

Date

Time

Venue

Theme/Focus:

Props

Oils

Music

No. Of
Attendees:

Private class: y / n

Note

-
-
-
-
-
-
-
-

Feedback

☆ ☆ ☆ ☆ ☆

Mantra / Positive Quote:

Yoga Teacher Planner

Date

Time

Venue

Theme/Focus:

Props . . . .

Oils

Music

No. Of Attendees:

Private class: y / n

Note

○
○
○
○
○
○
○
○

Feedback

☆ ☆ ☆ ☆ ☆

Mantra / Positive Quote:

Yoga Teacher Planner

Date

Time

Venue

Theme/Focus:

Props

Oils

Music

No. Of
Attendees:

Private class: y / n

Note

○
○
○
○
○
○
○
○

Feedback

☆ ☆ ☆ ☆ ☆

Mantra / Positive Quote:

Yoga Teacher Planner

Date

Time

Venue

Theme/Focus:

Props

Oils

Music

No. Of Attendees:

Private class: y / n

Note

-
-
-
-
-
-
-
-

Feedback

☆ ☆ ☆ ☆ ☆

Mantra / Positive Quote:

Yoga Teacher Planner

Date

Time

Venue

Theme/Focus:

Props

Oils

Music

No. Of
Attendees:

Private class: y / n

Note

○
○
○
○
○
○
○
○

Feedback

☆ ☆ ☆ ☆ ☆

Mantra / Positive Quote:

Yoga Teacher Planner

Date

Time

Venue

Theme/Focus:

Props

Oils

Music

No. Of
Attendees:

Private class: y / n

Note

○
○
○
○
○
○
○
○

Feedback

☆ ☆ ☆ ☆ ☆

Mantra / Positive Quote:

Yoga Teacher Planner

Date

Time

Venue

Theme/Focus:

Props

Oils

Music

No. Of
Attendees:

Private class: y / n

Note

○
○
○
○
○
○
○
○

Feedback

☆ ☆ ☆ ☆ ☆

Mantra / Positive Quote:

Yoga Teacher Planner

Date

Time

Venue

Theme/Focus:

Props

Oils

Music

No. Of
Attendees:

Private class: y / n

Note

Feedback

☆ ☆ ☆ ☆ ☆

Mantra / Positive Quote:

Yoga Teacher Planner

Date

Time

Venue

Theme/Focus:

Props

Oils

Music

No. Of
Attendees:

Private class: y / n

Note

○
○
○
○
○
○
○
○

Feedback

☆ ☆ ☆ ☆ ☆

Mantra / Positive Quote:

Yoga Teacher Planner

Date

Time

Venue

Theme/Focus:

Props

Oils

Music

No. Of Attendees:

Private class: y / n

Note

Feedback

☆ ☆ ☆ ☆ ☆

Mantra / Positive Quote:

Yoga Teacher Planner

Date

Time

Venue

Theme/Focus:

Props

Oils

Music

No. Of
Attendees:

Private class: y / n

Note

Feedback

☆ ☆ ☆ ☆ ☆

Mantra / Positive Quote:

Yoga Teacher Planner

Date

Time

Venue

Theme/Focus:

Props

. . . .
. . . .
. . . .
. . . .
. . . .
. . . .
. . . .
. . . .
. . . .
. . . .

Oils   Music

No. Of
Attendees:

Private class: y / n

Note

○ ______________
○ ______________
○ ______________
○ ______________
○ ______________
○ ______________
○ ______________
○ ______________

Feedback

☆ ☆ ☆ ☆ ☆

Mantra / Positive Quote:

Yoga Teacher Planner

Date

Time

Venue

Theme/Focus:

Props

Oils

Music

No. Of Attendees:

Private class: y / n

Note

- ○
- ○
- ○
- ○
- ○
- ○
- ○
- ○

Feedback

☆ ☆ ☆ ☆ ☆

Mantra / Positive Quote:

Yoga Teacher Planner

Date

Time

Venue

Theme/Focus:

Props

Oils

Music

No. Of Attendees:

Private class: y / n

Note

○
○
○
○
○
○
○
○

Feedback

☆ ☆ ☆ ☆ ☆

Mantra / Positive Quote:

Yoga Teacher Planner

Date

Time

Venue

Theme/Focus:

Props

. . . .

Oils

Music

No. Of
Attendees:

Private class: y / n

Note

○
○
○
○
○
○
○
○

Feedback

☆ ☆ ☆ ☆ ☆

Mantra / Positive Quote:

Yoga Teacher Planner

Date

Time

Venue

Theme/Focus:

Props

Oils

Music

No. Of
Attendees:

Private class: y / n

Note

- ○
- ○
- ○
- ○
- ○
- ○
- ○
- ○

Feedback

☆ ☆ ☆ ☆ ☆

Mantra / Positive Quote:

Yoga Teacher Planner

Date

Time

Venue

Theme/Focus:

Props

Oils

Music

No. Of
Attendees:

Private class: y / n

Note

- ○
- ○
- ○
- ○
- ○
- ○
- ○
- ○

Feedback

☆ ☆ ☆ ☆ ☆

Mantra / Positive Quote:

Yoga Teacher Planner

Date

Time

Venue

Theme/Focus:

Props . . . .

Oils   **Music**

No. Of Attendees:

Private class: y / n

Note

○
○
○
○
○
○
○
○

Feedback

☆ ☆ ☆ ☆ ☆

Mantra / Positive Quote:

Yoga Teacher Planner

Date ....

Time ....

Venue ....

Theme/Focus: ....

Props

Oils

Music

No. Of
Attendees: ....

Private class: y / n

Note

- ○ ___________________
- ○ ___________________
- ○ ___________________
- ○ ___________________
- ○ ___________________
- ○ ___________________
- ○ ___________________
- ○ ___________________

Feedback

☆ ☆ ☆ ☆ ☆

Mantra / Positive Quote:

Yoga Teacher Planner

Date

Time

Venue

Theme/Focus:

Props

Oils

Music

No. Of Attendees:

Private class: y / n

Note

Feedback

☆ ☆ ☆ ☆ ☆

Mantra / Positive Quote:

Yoga Teacher Planner

Date

Time

Venue

Theme/Focus:

Props

Oils

Music

No. Of Attendees:

Private class: y / n

Note

○
○
○
○
○
○
○
○

Feedback

☆ ☆ ☆ ☆ ☆

Mantra / Positive Quote:

Yoga Teacher Planner

Date

Time

Venue

Theme/Focus:

Props

Oils

Music

No. Of
Attendees:

Private class: y / n

Note

○
○
○
○
○
○
○
○
○

Feedback

☆ ☆ ☆ ☆ ☆

Mantra / Positive Quote:

Yoga Teacher Planner

Date

Time

Venue

Theme/Focus:

Props

Oils

Music

No. Of
Attendees:

Private class: y / n

Note

○
○
○
○
○
○
○
○

Feedback

☆ ☆ ☆ ☆ ☆

Mantra / Positive Quote:

Yoga Teacher Planner

Date

Time

Venue

Theme/Focus:

Props

Oils

Music

No. Of Attendees:

Private class: y / n

Note

- ○
- ○
- ○
- ○
- ○
- ○
- ○
- ○

Feedback

☆ ☆ ☆ ☆ ☆

Mantra / Positive Quote:

Yoga Teacher Planner

Date

Time

Venue

Theme/Focus:

Props

Oils

Music

No. Of Attendees:

Private class: y / n

Note

○
○
○
○
○
○
○
○

Feedback

☆ ☆ ☆ ☆ ☆

Mantra / Positive Quote:

Yoga Teacher Planner

Date

Time

Venue

Theme/Focus:

Props

Oils

Music

No. Of
Attendees:

Private class: y / n

Note

- ○
- ○
- ○
- ○
- ○
- ○
- ○
- ○

Feedback

☆ ☆ ☆ ☆ ☆

Mantra / Positive Quote:

Yoga Teacher Planner

Date

Time

Venue

Theme/Focus:

Props

Oils

Music

No. Of
Attendees:

Private class: y / n

Note

○
○
○
○
○
○
○
○

Feedback

☆ ☆ ☆ ☆ ☆

Mantra / Positive Quote:

Yoga Teacher Planner

Date

Time

Venue

Theme/Focus:

Props

Oils

Music

No. Of Attendees:

Private class: y / n

Note

Feedback

☆ ☆ ☆ ☆ ☆

Mantra / Positive Quote:

Yoga Teacher Planner

Date

Time

Venue

Theme/Focus:

Props

Oils

Music

No. Of
Attendees:

Private class: y / n

Note

○
○
○
○
○
○
○
○

Feedback

☆ ☆ ☆ ☆ ☆

Mantra / Positive Quote:

Yoga Teacher Planner

Date

Time

Venue

Theme/Focus:

Props . . . .

Oils

Music

No. Of Attendees:

Private class: y / n

Note

○
○
○
○
○
○
○
○

Feedback

☆ ☆ ☆ ☆ ☆

Mantra / Positive Quote:

Yoga Teacher Planner

Date

Time

Venue

Theme/Focus:

Props

Oils

Music

No. Of

Attendees:

Private class: y / n

Note

○
○
○
○
○
○
○
○

Feedback

☆ ☆ ☆ ☆ ☆

Mantra / Positive Quote:

Yoga Teacher Planner

Date

Time

Venue

Theme/Focus:

Props

Oils

Music

No. Of Attendees:

Private class: y / n

Note

Feedback

☆ ☆ ☆ ☆ ☆

Mantra / Positive Quote:

Yoga Teacher Planner

Date

Time

Venue

Theme/Focus:

Props

Oils

Music

No. Of
Attendees:

Private class: y / n

Note

- ○
- ○
- ○
- ○
- ○
- ○
- ○
- ○

Feedback

☆ ☆ ☆ ☆ ☆

Mantra / Positive Quote:

Yoga Teacher Planner

Date

Time

Venue

Theme/Focus:

Props

Oils

Music

No. Of Attendees:

Private class: y / n

Note

- ◯
- ◯
- ◯
- ◯
- ◯
- ◯
- ◯
- ◯

Feedback

☆ ☆ ☆ ☆ ☆

Mantra / Positive Quote:

Yoga Teacher Planner

Date

Time

Venue

Theme/Focus:

Props

Oils

Music

No. Of
Attendees:

Private class: y / n

Note

○
○
○
○
○
○
○
○

Feedback

☆ ☆ ☆ ☆ ☆

Mantra / Positive Quote:

Yoga Teacher Planner

Date

Time

Venue

Theme/Focus:

Props

Oils

Music

No. Of Attendees:

Private class: y / n

Note

- ○
- ○
- ○
- ○
- ○
- ○
- ○
- ○

Feedback

☆ ☆ ☆ ☆ ☆

Mantra / Positive Quote:

Yoga Teacher Planner

Date

Time

Venue

Theme/Focus:

Props

Oils

Music

No. Of Attendees:

Private class: y / n

Note

- ○
- ○
- ○
- ○
- ○
- ○
- ○
- ○

Feedback

☆ ☆ ☆ ☆ ☆

Mantra / Positive Quote:

Yoga Teacher Planner

Date

Time

Venue

Theme/Focus:

Props . . . .

Oils

Music

No. Of
Attendees:

Private class: y / n

Note

○
○
○
○
○
○
○
○

Feedback

☆ ☆ ☆ ☆ ☆

Mantra / Positive Quote:

Yoga Teacher Planner

Date

Time

Venue

Theme/Focus:

Props

Oils

Music

No. Of Attendees:

Private class: y / n

Note

○
○
○
○
○
○
○
○

Feedback

☆ ☆ ☆ ☆ ☆

Mantra / Positive Quote:

Yoga Teacher Planner

Date

Time

Venue

Theme/Focus:

Props

Oils

Music

No. Of Attendees:

Private class: y / n

Note

○
○
○
○
○
○
○
○

Feedback

☆ ☆ ☆ ☆ ☆

Mantra / Positive Quote:

Yoga Teacher Planner

Date

Time

Venue

Theme/Focus:

Props

Oils

Music

No. Of
Attendees:

Private class: y / n

Note

Feedback

☆ ☆ ☆ ☆ ☆

Mantra / Positive Quote:

Yoga Teacher Planner

Date

Time

Venue

Theme/Focus:

Props

Oils

Music

No. Of Attendees:

Private class: y / n

Note

- ○
- ○
- ○
- ○
- ○
- ○
- ○
- ○

Feedback

☆ ☆ ☆ ☆ ☆

Mantra / Positive Quote:

Yoga Teacher Planner

Date

Time

Venue

Theme/Focus:

Props

Oils

Music

No. Of
Attendees:

Private class: y / n

Note

○
○
○
○
○
○
○
○

Feedback

☆ ☆ ☆ ☆ ☆

Mantra / Positive Quote:

Yoga Teacher Planner

Date

Time

Venue

Theme/Focus:

Props . . . .
. . . .
. . . .
. . . .
. . . .
. . . .
. . . .
. . . .
. . . .
. . . .
. . . .

Oils   **Music**

No. Of Attendees:

Private class: y / n

Note

○ ________________
○ ________________
○ ________________
○ ________________
○ ________________
○ ________________
○ ________________
○ ________________

Feedback

☆ ☆ ☆ ☆ ☆

Mantra / Positive Quote:

Yoga Teacher Planner

Date

Time

Venue

Theme/Focus:

Props

Oils

Music

No. Of Attendees:

Private class: y / n

Note

○
○
○
○
○
○
○
○

Feedback

☆ ☆ ☆ ☆ ☆

Mantra / Positive Quote:

Yoga Teacher Planner

Date

Time

Venue

Theme/Focus:

Props . . . .
. . . .
. . . .
. . . .
. . . .
. . . .
. . . .
. . . .
. . . .
. . . .
. . . .

Oils

Music

No. Of Attendees:

Private class: y / n

Note

○
○
○
○
○
○
○
○
○

Feedback

☆ ☆ ☆ ☆ ☆

Mantra / Positive Quote:

Yoga Teacher Planner

Date

Time

Venue

Theme/Focus:

Props

Oils

Music

No. Of
Attendees:

Private class: y / n

Note

- ○
- ○
- ○
- ○
- ○
- ○
- ○
- ○

Feedback

☆ ☆ ☆ ☆ ☆

Mantra / Positive Quote:

Yoga Teacher Planner

Date

Time

Venue

Theme/Focus:

Props

Oils

Music

No. Of
Attendees:

Private class: y / n

Note

- ○
- ○
- ○
- ○
- ○
- ○
- ○
- ○

Feedback

☆ ☆ ☆ ☆ ☆

Mantra / Positive Quote:

Yoga Teacher Planner

Date

Time

Venue

Theme/Focus:

Props

Oils

Music

No. Of Attendees:

Private class: y / n

Note

- ○
- ○
- ○
- ○
- ○
- ○
- ○
- ○

Feedback

☆ ☆ ☆ ☆ ☆

Mantra / Positive Quote:

Yoga Teacher Planner

Date

Time

Venue

Theme/Focus:

Props

Oils

Music

No. Of
Attendees:

Private class: y / n

Note

○
○
○
○
○
○
○
○

Feedback

☆ ☆ ☆ ☆ ☆

Mantra / Positive Quote:

Yoga Teacher Planner

Date

Time

Venue

Theme/Focus:

Props

Oils

Music

No. Of
Attendees:

Private class: y / n

Note

○
○
○
○
○
○
○
○

Feedback

☆ ☆ ☆ ☆ ☆

Mantra / Positive Quote:

Yoga Teacher Planner

Date

Time

Venue

Theme/Focus:

Props

Oils

Music

No. Of
Attendees:

Private class: y / n

Note

○
○
○
○
○
○
○
○

Feedback

☆ ☆ ☆ ☆ ☆

Mantra / Positive Quote:

Yoga Teacher Planner

Date ....

Time ....

Venue ....

Theme/Focus: ....

Props

Oils

Music

No. Of Attendees: ....

Private class: y / n

Note

- ○ ....
- ○ ....
- ○ ....
- ○ ....
- ○ ....
- ○ ....
- ○ ....
- ○ ....

Feedback

☆ ☆ ☆ ☆ ☆

Mantra / Positive Quote:

Yoga Teacher Planner

Date

Time

Venue

Theme/Focus:

Props

Oils

Music

No. Of Attendees:

Private class: y / n

Note

Feedback

☆ ☆ ☆ ☆ ☆

Mantra / Positive Quote:

Yoga Teacher Planner

Date

Time

Venue

Theme/Focus:

Props

Oils

Music

No. Of
Attendees:

Private class: y / n

Note

- ○
- ○
- ○
- ○
- ○
- ○
- ○
- ○

Feedback

☆ ☆ ☆ ☆ ☆

Mantra / Positive Quote:

Yoga Teacher Planner

Date

Time

Venue

Theme/Focus:

Props

Oils

Music

No. Of Attendees:

Private class: y / n

Note

- ○
- ○
- ○
- ○
- ○
- ○
- ○
- ○

Feedback

☆ ☆ ☆ ☆ ☆

Mantra / Positive Quote:

Yoga Teacher Planner

Date

Time

Venue

Theme/Focus:

Props

Oils

Music

No. Of Attendees:

Private class: y / n

Note

- ○
- ○
- ○
- ○
- ○
- ○
- ○
- ○

Feedback

☆ ☆ ☆ ☆ ☆

Mantra / Positive Quote:

Yoga Teacher Planner

Date

Time

Venue

Theme/Focus:

Props . . . .

Oils

Music

No. Of
Attendees:

Private class: y / n

Note

○
○
○
○
○
○
○
○

Feedback

☆ ☆ ☆ ☆ ☆

Mantra / Positive Quote:

Yoga Teacher Planner

Date

Time

Venue

Theme/Focus:

Props

Oils

Music

No. Of
Attendees:

Private class: y / n

Note

- ○
- ○
- ○
- ○
- ○
- ○
- ○
- ○

Feedback

☆ ☆ ☆ ☆ ☆

Mantra / Positive Quote:

Yoga Teacher Planner

Date

Time

Venue

Theme/Focus:

Props

Oils

Music

No. Of Attendees:

Private class: y / n

Note

- ○
- ○
- ○
- ○
- ○
- ○
- ○
- ○

Feedback

☆ ☆ ☆ ☆ ☆

Mantra / Positive Quote:

Yoga Teacher Planner

Date

Time

Venue

Theme/Focus:

Props

Oils

Music

No. Of Attendees:

Private class: y / n

Note

○
○
○
○
○
○
○
○

Feedback

☆ ☆ ☆ ☆ ☆

Mantra / Positive Quote:

Yoga Teacher Planner

Date

Time

Venue

Theme/Focus:

Props

Oils

Music

No. Of Attendees:

Private class: y / n

Note

Feedback

☆ ☆ ☆ ☆ ☆

Mantra / Positive Quote:

Yoga Teacher Planner

Date

Time

Venue

Theme/Focus:

Props

Oils

Music

No. Of Attendees:

Private class: y / n

Note

Feedback

☆ ☆ ☆ ☆ ☆

Mantra / Positive Quote:

Yoga Teacher Planner

Date

Time

Venue

Theme/Focus:

Props . . . .

Oils

Music

No. Of Attendees:

Private class: y / n

Note

○
○
○
○
○
○
○
○

Feedback

☆ ☆ ☆ ☆ ☆

Mantra / Positive Quote:

Yoga Teacher Planner

Date

Time

Venue

Theme/Focus:

Props

Oils

Music

No. Of
Attendees:

Private class: y / n

Note

○
○
○
○
○
○
○
○

Feedback

☆ ☆ ☆ ☆ ☆

Mantra / Positive Quote:

Yoga Teacher Planner

Date

Time

Venue

Theme/Focus:

Props

Oils

Music

No. Of Attendees:

Private class: y / n

Note

Feedback

☆ ☆ ☆ ☆ ☆

Mantra / Positive Quote:

Yoga Teacher Planner

Date

Time

Venue

Theme/Focus:

Props

Oils

Music

No. Of Attendees:

Private class: y / n

Note

○
○
○
○
○
○
○
○

Feedback

☆ ☆ ☆ ☆ ☆

Mantra / Positive Quote:

Yoga Teacher Planner

Date

Time

Venue

Theme/Focus:

Props

Oils

Music

No. Of
Attendees:

Private class: y / n

Note

○
○
○
○
○
○
○
○

Feedback

☆ ☆ ☆ ☆ ☆

Mantra / Positive Quote:

Yoga Teacher Planner

Date

Time

Venue

Theme/Focus:

Props

Oils

Music

No. Of
Attendees:

Private class: y / n

Note

- ○
- ○
- ○
- ○
- ○
- ○
- ○
- ○

Feedback

☆ ☆ ☆ ☆ ☆

Mantra / Positive Quote:

Yoga Teacher Planner

Date

Time

Venue

Theme/Focus:

Props

Oils

Music

No. Of Attendees:

Private class: y / n

Note

- ○
- ○
- ○
- ○
- ○
- ○
- ○
- ○

Feedback

☆ ☆ ☆ ☆ ☆

Mantra / Positive Quote:

Yoga Teacher Planner

Date

Time

Venue

Theme/Focus:

Props

Oils

Music

No. Of
Attendees:

Private class: y / n

Note

○
○
○
○
○
○
○
○

Feedback

☆ ☆ ☆ ☆ ☆

Mantra / Positive Quote:

Yoga Teacher Planner

Date

Time

Venue

Theme/Focus:

Props

Oils

Music

No. Of
Attendees:

Private class: y / n

Note

- ○
- ○
- ○
- ○
- ○
- ○
- ○
- ○

Feedback

☆ ☆ ☆ ☆ ☆

Mantra / Positive Quote:

Yoga Teacher Planner

Date

Time

Venue

Theme/Focus:

Props

Oils

Music

No. Of Attendees:

Private class: y / n

Note

○
○
○
○
○
○
○
○

Feedback

☆ ☆ ☆ ☆ ☆

Mantra / Positive Quote:

Yoga Teacher Planner

Date

Time

Venue

Theme/Focus:

Props . . . .

Oils

Music

No. Of
Attendees:

Private class: y / n

Note

- ○
- ○
- ○
- ○
- ○
- ○
- ○
- ○

Feedback

☆ ☆ ☆ ☆ ☆

Mantra / Positive Quote:

Yoga Teacher Planner

Date

Time

Venue

Theme/Focus:

Props

Oils

Music

No. Of
Attendees:

Private class: y / n

Note

- ◯
- ◯
- ◯
- ◯
- ◯
- ◯
- ◯
- ◯

Feedback

☆ ☆ ☆ ☆ ☆

Mantra / Positive Quote:

Yoga Teacher Planner

Date

Time

Venue

Theme/Focus:

Props

Oils

Music

No. Of
Attendees:

Private class: y / n

Note

Feedback

☆ ☆ ☆ ☆ ☆

Mantra / Positive Quote:

Yoga Teacher Planner

Date

Time

Venue

Theme/Focus:

Props

Oils

Music

No. Of
Attendees:

Private class: y / n

Note

○
○
○
○
○
○
○
○

Feedback

☆ ☆ ☆ ☆ ☆

Mantra / Positive Quote:

Yoga Teacher Planner

Date

Time

Venue

Theme/Focus:

Props

Oils

Music

No. Of Attendees:

Private class: y / n

Note

- ○
- ○
- ○
- ○
- ○
- ○
- ○
- ○

Feedback

☆ ☆ ☆ ☆ ☆

Mantra / Positive Quote:

Yoga Teacher Planner

Date

Time

Venue

Theme/Focus:

Props

Oils

Music

No. Of Attendees:

Private class: y / n

Note

- ○
- ○
- ○
- ○
- ○
- ○
- ○
- ○

Feedback

☆ ☆ ☆ ☆ ☆

Mantra / Positive Quote:

Yoga Teacher Planner

Date

Time

Venue

Theme/Focus:

Props

Oils

Music

No. Of Attendees:

Private class: y / n

Note

○ _______________
○ _______________
○ _______________
○ _______________
○ _______________
○ _______________
○ _______________
○ _______________

Feedback

☆ ☆ ☆ ☆ ☆

Mantra / Positive Quote:

Yoga Teacher Planner

Date

Time

Venue

Theme/Focus:

Props

Oils

Music

No. Of Attendees:

Private class: y / n

Note

- ○
- ○
- ○
- ○
- ○
- ○
- ○
- ○

Feedback

☆ ☆ ☆ ☆ ☆

Mantra / Positive Quote:

Yoga Teacher Planner

Date

Time

Venue

Theme/Focus:

Props

Oils

Music

No. Of Attendees:

Private class: y / n

Note

○
○
○
○
○
○
○
○
○

Feedback

☆ ☆ ☆ ☆ ☆

Mantra / Positive Quote:

Yoga Teacher Planner

Date

Time

Venue

Theme/Focus:

Props

Oils

Music

No. Of Attendees:

Private class: y / n

Note

- ◯
- ◯
- ◯
- ◯
- ◯
- ◯
- ◯
- ◯

Feedback

☆ ☆ ☆ ☆ ☆

Mantra / Positive Quote:

Yoga Teacher Planner

Date

Time

Venue

Theme/Focus:

Props

Oils

Music

No. Of Attendees:

Private class: y / n

Note

- ○
- ○
- ○
- ○
- ○
- ○
- ○
- ○

Feedback

☆ ☆ ☆ ☆ ☆

Mantra / Positive Quote:

Yoga Teacher Planner

Date

Time

Venue

Theme/Focus:

Props

Oils

Music

No. Of
Attendees:

Private class: y / n

Note

○
○
○
○
○
○
○
○

Feedback

☆ ☆ ☆ ☆ ☆

Mantra / Positive Quote:

Yoga Teacher Planner

Date

Time

Venue

Theme/Focus:

Props

Oils

Music

No. Of
Attendees:

Private class: y / n

Note

○
○
○
○
○
○
○
○

Feedback

☆ ☆ ☆ ☆ ☆

Mantra / Positive Quote:

Yoga Teacher Planner

Date

Time

Venue

Theme/Focus:

Props

Oils

Music

No. Of Attendees:

Private class: y / n

Note

- ○
- ○
- ○
- ○
- ○
- ○
- ○
- ○

Feedback

☆ ☆ ☆ ☆ ☆

Mantra / Positive Quote:

Yoga Teacher Planner

Date

Time

Venue

Theme/Focus:

Props

Oils

Music

No. Of
Attendees:

Private class: y / n

Note

○ ____________
○ ____________
○ ____________
○ ____________
○ ____________
○ ____________
○ ____________
○ ____________

Feedback

☆ ☆ ☆ ☆ ☆

Mantra / Positive Quote:

Yoga Teacher Planner

Date

Time

Venue

Theme/Focus:

Props

Oils

Music

No. Of Attendees:

Private class: y / n

Note

- ○
- ○
- ○
- ○
- ○
- ○
- ○
- ○

Feedback

☆ ☆ ☆ ☆ ☆

Mantra / Positive Quote:

Yoga Teacher Planner

Date

Time

Venue

Theme/Focus:

Props

Oils

Music

No. Of
Attendees:

Private class: y / n

Note

○
○
○
○
○
○
○
○

Feedback

☆ ☆ ☆ ☆ ☆

Mantra / Positive Quote:

Yoga Teacher Planner

Date

Time

Venue

Theme/Focus:

Props

Oils

Music

No. Of Attendees:

Private class: y / n

Note

○
○
○
○
○
○
○
○

Feedback

☆ ☆ ☆ ☆ ☆

Mantra / Positive Quote:

Yoga Teacher Planner

Date

Time

Venue

Theme/Focus:

Props

. . . .
. . . .
. . . .
. . . .
. . . .
. . . .
. . . .
. . . .
. . . .

Oils

Music

No. Of Attendees:

Private class: y / n

Note

○ _____________
○ _____________
○ _____________
○ _____________
○ _____________
○ _____________
○ _____________
○ _____________

Feedback

☆ ☆ ☆ ☆ ☆

Mantra / Positive Quote:

Yoga Teacher Planner

Date

Time

Venue

Theme/Focus:

Props

Oils

Music

No. Of
Attendees:

Private class: y / n

Note

○
○
○
○
○
○
○
○

Feedback

☆ ☆ ☆ ☆ ☆

Mantra / Positive Quote:

Yoga Teacher Planner

Date

Time

Venue

Theme/Focus:

Props

Oils

Music

No. Of Attendees:

Private class: y / n

Note

○
○
○
○
○
○
○
○

Feedback

☆ ☆ ☆ ☆ ☆

Mantra / Positive Quote:

Yoga Teacher Planner

Date

Time

Venue

Theme/Focus:

Props

Oils

Music

No. Of
Attendees:

Private class: y / n

Note

- ◯
- ◯
- ◯
- ◯
- ◯
- ◯
- ◯
- ◯

Feedback

☆ ☆ ☆ ☆ ☆

Mantra / Positive Quote:

Yoga Teacher Planner

Date

Time

Venue

Theme/Focus:

Props

Oils

Music

No. Of Attendees:

Private class: y / n

Note

○
○
○
○
○
○
○
○

Feedback

☆ ☆ ☆ ☆ ☆

Mantra / Positive Quote:

Yoga Teacher Planner

Date

Time

Venue

Theme/Focus:

Props

Oils

Music

No. Of Attendees:

Private class: y / n

Note

- ○
- ○
- ○
- ○
- ○
- ○
- ○
- ○

Feedback

☆ ☆ ☆ ☆ ☆

Mantra / Positive Quote:

Yoga Teacher Planner

Date

Time

Venue

Theme/Focus:

Props

Oils

Music

No. Of
Attendees:

Private class: y / n

Note

○
○
○
○
○
○
○
○

Feedback

☆ ☆ ☆ ☆ ☆

Mantra / Positive Quote:

Yoga Teacher Planner

Date

Time

Venue

Theme/Focus:

Props

Oils

Music

No. Of
Attendees:

Private class: y / n

Note

- ◯
- ◯
- ◯
- ◯
- ◯
- ◯
- ◯
- ◯

Feedback

☆ ☆ ☆ ☆ ☆

Mantra / Positive Quote:

Yoga Teacher Planner

Date

Time

Venue

Theme/Focus:

Props

Oils

Music

No. Of
Attendees:

Private class: y / n

Note

-
-
-
-
-
-
-
-
-

Feedback

☆ ☆ ☆ ☆ ☆

Mantra / Positive Quote:

Yoga Teacher Planner

Date

Time

Venue

Theme/Focus:

Props

Oils

Music

No. Of Attendees:

Private class: y / n

Note

- ○
- ○
- ○
- ○
- ○
- ○
- ○
- ○

Feedback

☆ ☆ ☆ ☆ ☆

Mantra / Positive Quote:

Yoga Teacher Planner

Date

Time

Venue

Theme/Focus:

Props

Oils

Music

No. Of Attendees:

Private class: y / n

Note

-
-
-
-
-
-
-
-

Feedback

☆ ☆ ☆ ☆ ☆

Mantra / Positive Quote:

Yoga Teacher Planner

Date

Time

Venue

Theme/Focus:

Props

Oils

Music

No. Of Attendees:

Private class: y / n

Note

- ○
- ○
- ○
- ○
- ○
- ○
- ○
- ○

Feedback

☆ ☆ ☆ ☆ ☆

Mantra / Positive Quote:

Yoga Teacher Planner

Date

Time

Venue

Theme/Focus:

Props

Oils

Music

No. Of Attendees:

Private class: y / n

Note

○
○
○
○
○
○
○
○

Feedback

☆ ☆ ☆ ☆ ☆

Mantra / Positive Quote:

Yoga Teacher Planner

Date

Time

Venue

Theme/Focus:

Props

Oils

Music

No. Of Attendees:

Private class: y / n

Note

○
○
○
○
○
○
○
○

Feedback

☆ ☆ ☆ ☆ ☆

Mantra / Positive Quote:

Yoga Teacher Planner

Date

Time

Venue

Theme/Focus:

Props

Oils

Music

No. Of
Attendees:

Private class: y / n

Note

○
○
○
○
○
○
○
○

Feedback

☆ ☆ ☆ ☆ ☆

Mantra / Positive Quote:

Yoga Teacher Planner

Date

Time

Venue

Theme/Focus:

Props

Oils

Music

No. Of Attendees:

Private class: y / n

Note

- ○
- ○
- ○
- ○
- ○
- ○
- ○
- ○

Feedback

☆ ☆ ☆ ☆ ☆

Mantra / Positive Quote:

Yoga Teacher Planner

Date

Time

Venue

Theme/Focus:

Props

Oils

Music

No. Of Attendees:

Private class: y / n

Note

- ○
- ○
- ○
- ○
- ○
- ○
- ○
- ○

Feedback

☆ ☆ ☆ ☆ ☆

Mantra / Positive Quote:

Yoga Teacher Planner

Date

Time

Venue

Theme/Focus:

Props

Oils

Music

No. Of
Attendees:

Private class: y / n

Note

- ○
- ○
- ○
- ○
- ○
- ○
- ○
- ○

Feedback

☆ ☆ ☆ ☆ ☆

Mantra / Positive Quote:

Yoga Teacher Planner

Date

Time

Venue

Theme/Focus:

Props

Oils

Music

No. Of Attendees:

Private class: y / n

Note

- ○
- ○
- ○
- ○
- ○
- ○
- ○
- ○

Feedback

☆ ☆ ☆ ☆ ☆

Mantra / Positive Quote:

Yoga Teacher Planner

Date ....

Time ....

Venue ....

Theme/Focus: ....
....
....

Props ....

Oils

Music

No. Of Attendees: ....

Private class: y / n

Note

- ○ ———————————
- ○ ———————————
- ○ ———————————
- ○ ———————————
- ○ ———————————
- ○ ———————————
- ○ ———————————
- ○ ———————————

Feedback

☆ ☆ ☆ ☆ ☆

Mantra / Positive Quote:

Yoga Teacher Planner

Date

Time

Venue

Theme/Focus:

Props

Oils

Music

No. Of Attendees:

Private class: y / n

Note

Feedback

☆ ☆ ☆ ☆ ☆

Mantra / Positive Quote:

Yoga Teacher Planner

Date

Time

Venue

Theme/Focus:

Props

Oils

Music

No. Of
Attendees:

Private class: y / n

Note

Feedback

☆ ☆ ☆ ☆ ☆

Mantra / Positive Quote:

Yoga Teacher Planner

Date

Time

Venue

Theme/Focus:

Props

Oils

Music

No. Of Attendees:

Private class: y / n

Note

- ○
- ○
- ○
- ○
- ○
- ○
- ○
- ○

Feedback

☆ ☆ ☆ ☆ ☆

Mantra / Positive Quote:

Yoga Teacher Planner

Date

Time

Venue

Theme/Focus:

Props

Oils

Music

No. Of
Attendees:

Private class: y / n

Note

- ○
- ○
- ○
- ○
- ○
- ○
- ○
- ○

Feedback

☆ ☆ ☆ ☆ ☆

Mantra / Positive Quote:

Yoga Teacher Planner

Date

Time

Venue

Theme/Focus:

Props

Oils

Music

No. Of Attendees:

Private class: y / n

Note

- ○
- ○
- ○
- ○
- ○
- ○
- ○
- ○

Feedback

☆ ☆ ☆ ☆ ☆

Mantra / Positive Quote:

Yoga Teacher Planner

Date

Time

Venue

Theme/Focus:

Props

Oils

Music

No. Of
Attendees:

Private class: y / n

Note

Feedback

☆ ☆ ☆ ☆ ☆

Mantra / Positive Quote:

Yoga Teacher Planner

Date

Time

Venue

Theme/Focus:

Props . . . .

Oils

Music

No. Of
Attendees:

Private class: y / n

Note

- ○
- ○
- ○
- ○
- ○
- ○
- ○
- ○

Feedback

☆ ☆ ☆ ☆ ☆

Mantra / Positive Quote:

Yoga Teacher Planner

Date

Time

Venue

Theme/Focus:

Props

Oils

Music

No. Of
Attendees:

Private class: y / n

Note

○
○
○
○
○
○
○
○

Feedback

☆ ☆ ☆ ☆ ☆

Mantra / Positive Quote:

Yoga Teacher Planner

Date

Time

Venue

Theme/Focus:

Props

. . . .

Oils

Music

No. Of
Attendees:

Private class: y / n

Note

○
○
○
○
○
○
○
○

Feedback

☆ ☆ ☆ ☆ ☆

Mantra / Positive Quote:

Yoga Teacher Planner

Date

Time

Venue

Theme/Focus:

Props

Oils

Music

No. Of Attendees:

Private class: y / n

Note

○
○
○
○
○
○
○
○

Feedback

☆ ☆ ☆ ☆ ☆

Mantra / Positive Quote:

Yoga Teacher Planner

Date

Time

Venue

Theme/Focus:

Props

Oils

Music

No. Of Attendees:

Private class: y / n

Note

○
○
○
○
○
○
○
○

Feedback

☆ ☆ ☆ ☆ ☆

Mantra / Positive Quote:

Yoga Teacher Planner

Date

Time

Venue

Theme/Focus:

Props

Oils

Music

No. Of Attendees:

Private class: y / n

Note

- ○
- ○
- ○
- ○
- ○
- ○
- ○
- ○

Feedback

☆ ☆ ☆ ☆ ☆

Mantra / Positive Quote:

Yoga Teacher Planner

Date

Time

Venue

Theme/Focus:

Props

Oils

Music

No. Of Attendees:

Private class: y / n

Note

- ○
- ○
- ○
- ○
- ○
- ○
- ○
- ○

Feedback

☆ ☆ ☆ ☆ ☆

Mantra / Positive Quote:

Yoga Teacher Planner

Date

Time

Venue

Theme/Focus:

Props

Oils

Music

No. Of Attendees:

Private class: y / n

Note

- ○
- ○
- ○
- ○
- ○
- ○
- ○
- ○

Feedback

☆ ☆ ☆ ☆ ☆

Mantra / Positive Quote:

Yoga Teacher Planner

Date

Time

Venue

Theme/Focus:

Props

Oils

Music

No. Of Attendees:

Private class: y / n

Note

Feedback

☆ ☆ ☆ ☆ ☆

Mantra / Positive Quote: